# Best Sex Toys for Long Distance Relationship

## 20+ Top Adult Sex Toys for Long Distance Couples – Vibrators, Dildos, and Accessories

Cheryl Bach

# Best Sex Toys for Long Distance Relationship

©2024 by Cheryl Bach



Publisher: IntimateInk Press

Email: intimateinkpress@gmail.com



Cover design by IntimateInk Press

Interior layout and design by IntimateInk Press

Printed in USA

Fonts: Google fonts

Image: Freepik.com. This cover has been designed using assets from Freepik.com

For permission to use copyrighted material from this book, please contact the copyright holder listed above.

First Edition: 2024

Distributed by Amazon.com, Inc.

Cheryl Bach

# Table of Contents

# Best Sex Toys for Long Distance Relationship

Cheryl Bach

# Introduction

As more and more couples are finding themselves in long distance relationships, it can be difficult to keep the spark alive when you're miles apart from your partner. That's where "Best Sex Toys for Long Distance Relationships: 20+ Top Adult Sex Toys for Long Distance Couples – Vibrators, Dildos, and Accessories" comes in.

This book is a necessity for anyone in a long distance relationship who wants to spice up their sex life and strengthen their connection with their partner. Many couples in long distance relationships are clueless on how to keep things exciting when they can't be together physically, but with the right tools, anything is possible.

Best Sex Toys for Long Distance Relationship

Inside this comprehensive guide, you'll discover 20+ of the best adult sex toys for long distance couples, including vibrators, dildos, and accessories. Each toy is carefully selected and reviewed, ensuring that you can trust that you're getting the best of the best.

With this book as your guide, you'll be able to explore new levels of intimacy and pleasure with your partner no matter where you are in the world. Whether you're looking to enhance your video chat sessions or simply want to add some excitement to your sexting sessions, there's a sex toy out there that's perfect for you.

Investing in the right sex toys for your long distance relationship can be a game-changer, and this book will help you navigate the often overwhelming world of adult toys so that you can choose ones that will truly enhance your connection with your partner.

Cheryl Bach

Get ready to take your intimate moments to the next level with "Best Sex Toys for Long Distance Relationships: 20+ Top Adult Sex Toys for Long Distance Couples – Vibrators, Dildos, and Accessories".

This book is a valuable resource that will not only help you find the perfect sex toy for your unique needs but also offer tips on how to use them effectively to add excitement and intimacy to your long-distance relationship. You'll also gain insights on how to communicate your desires with your partner and build trust and connection through virtual intimacy.

Don't let distance interfere with your physical and emotional needs. "Best Sex Toys for Long Distance Relationships" is here to guide you to finding the essential tools for enhancing and maintaining your relationship's satisfaction and spice, no matter the distance.

# Chapter 1

## Lovense Lush 2

Lovense Lush 2 is a wearable vibrator that is perfect for long distance couples. It is a highly advanced tech sex toy that uses Bluetooth technology to connect to a smartphone or tablet app. This app allows the wearer or their partner to control the device from anywhere in the world, making it an ideal choice for couples who are physically apart.

The Lovense Lush 2 is designed to be worn inside the vaginal canal and is perfect for hands-free solo-pleasure or for use during sexual activities with your partner. The device has several vibration patterns and intensities, all of which can be controlled from the app. This allows for complete customization of your experience and ensures that no two sessions are ever the same.

One of the most significant advantages of the Lovense Lush 2 is its unique design. The shape and size of the device make it incredibly discreet and comfortable to wear for extended periods, making it perfect for all-day use. This is particularly beneficial for long distance couples as it allows for a heightened level of intimacy throughout the day.

Furthermore, the Lovense Lush 2 has a long battery life, which means that it can be used for extended periods without needing to be recharged. This is especially useful during longer video chat sessions or when you know that you won't have access to a charging point for an extended period.

The Lovense Lush 2 is also made from high-quality, body-safe materials, which ensure that it is both hygienic and comfortable to wear. The device is also easy to clean and maintain, meaning that it can be used multiple times without any issues.

Overall, the Lovense Lush 2 is an excellent choice for long distance couples who are looking to enhance their intimate relationship. Its unique design, advanced technology, and customizable features make it a great pick for anyone looking to spice up their long distance experience.

Not only is the Lovense Lush 2 perfect for solo play, but it can also be used during virtual sex sessions with your partner. This allows for a more immersive experience and can help you feel closer to your partner, even when you're miles apart.

Moreover, the smartphone app that controls the device also allows for long distance couples to stay connected and communicate during their intimate moments. The app lets you send custom vibrations and messages to your partner, which creates a new level of intimacy, even when you're not physically together.

In conclusion, the Lovense Lush 2 is an incredible addition to any long distance couple's sex toy collection. Its customizable features, discreet design, and long battery life make it an excellent pick for those who are looking for an enhanced level of intimacy and connection in their long distance relationship. With the ability to control the device from anywhere in the world and the advanced technology that allows for a truly immersive experience, the Lovense Lush 2 is a must-try for anyone looking to stay connected with their partner, both emotionally and physically.

So whether you're a seasoned pro when it comes to sex toys or a first-time user, the Lovense Lush 2 is definitely worth considering. Its innovative design, high-quality materials, and customizable vibrations make it one of the best sex toys available for long distance couples today.

Don't let distance come in the way of your intimate relationship; invest in a Lovense Lush 2 today and start exploring new heights of pleasure and connection with your partner.

# Chapter 2

## Kiiroo Onyx+ & Pearl2 Couple Set

The Kiiroo Onyx+ and Pearl2 Couple Set is a unique sex toy kit designed for long distance couples. The set includes the Onyx+ male masturbator and the Pearl2 interactive vibrator, both of which are made to be used together to simulate sex from afar.

The Onyx+ is a high-tech male masturbator that uses realistic movements to create an immersive experience for the user. It can be controlled remotely via Bluetooth and has various vibration levels and patterns that can be customized to suit personal preferences.

On the other hand, the Pearl2 is a sleek and highly advanced vibrator that provides powerful stimulation and can also be controlled remotely using the companion Kiiroo app. This allows for real-time control and synchronization, which creates a truly immersive long distance experience for both partners.

When used together, the Kiiroo Onyx+ and Pearl2 create a realistic and intimate experience that can help long distance couples feel closer and more connected. The devices are designed to simulate the sensations of real intercourse, providing users with a lifelike experience that can help create a deeply satisfying sexual experience.

One of the key benefits of the Kiiroo Onyx+ and Pearl2 Couple Set is its ability to create a sense of mutual pleasure. When both devices are used at the same time, the vibrations and movements are synchronized, meaning that both partners can enjoy the same sensations at the same time, no matter how far apart they are.

Another significant advantage of this couple set is the level of customization that it offers. Users can choose from various vibration patterns and adjust the intensity levels according to their preferences. Additionally, the remote control feature allows for easy and discrete control, so users can enjoy a pleasurable experience without attracting unwanted attention.

Moreover, the Kiiroo Onyx+ and Pearl2 Couple Set is an excellent pick for long distance couples because it can help build trust and intimacy in a relationship. When partners are separated by distance, it can be challenging to maintain a deep emotional connection. However, by sharing intimate moments, even from afar, couples can strengthen their bond and deepen their understanding of one another.

The set has a sophisticated design that makes it easy to use and clean. The devices are made from high-quality, body-safe materials that ensure the user's health and safety. Additionally, the devices' discreet design makes them perfect for solo play, so users can enjoy the set without attracting unwanted attention.

Overall, the Kiiroo Onyx+ and Pearl2 Couple Set is an excellent investment for long distance couples who want to enhance their intimacy and connection. Its innovative design, customizable features and mutual stimulation capabilities make it stand out among other sex toys for long distance relationships. The use of high-tech technology and real-time synchronization ensures a genuinely immersive experience, providing users with an intimate and sensitive connection that is hard to replicate elsewhere.

In summary, the Kiiroo Onyx+ and Pearl2 Couple Set is in every way an exceptional choice of sex toy for couples in long distance relationships. By providing a sense of closeness and mutual pleasure, it helps overcome the physical boundaries that distance brings. It is not just a toy, but an essential part of intimacy and connection-building tool for long-distance partners. Investing in the couple's set is a game-changer for the well-being of the relationship, bringing joy and satisfaction beyond geographical locations.

# Chapter 3

## We-Vibe Sync

The We-Vibe Sync is a versatile sex toy designed for long-distance couples who seek to deepen their connection and enhance their intimacy. It is both a clitoral and G-spot vibrator that can be used during intercourse or solo play.

The Sync features an advanced design that allows it to be comfortably worn during sex. It is a hands-free device that provides dual stimulation, allowing users to experience intense, multiple orgasms. Additionally, its adjustable fit allows it to be tailored to each user's body shape, ensuring maximum comfort and pleasure.

One of the most significant advantages of the We-Vibe Sync is the convenience it offers for long distance couples. The device can be controlled remotely via the We-Connect app, allowing users to connect with one another and share intimate moments no matter where they are in the world.

The We-Connect app offers a myriad of customizable features that allow users to personalize their We-Vibe Sync experience. It provides a range of vibration patterns and intensity levels that can be modified according to personal preferences, making it an ideal stimulator for long, sensual sessions. The app also allows partners to control each other's device, providing a genuinely immersive experience that deepens emotional intimacy and builds trust.

Another great feature of the We-Vibe Sync is its ability to enhance couples intercourse. During sex, the Sync provides clitoral and G-spot stimulation, providing more intense orgasms for the user. Its compact design ensures that there is no interference with penetration, making it an excellent choice for couples looking to add extra spice to their intimate moments.

When it comes to long-distance relationships, the We-Vibe Sync makes a great pick because it provides couples with a unique level of sexual intimacy that can't be found with traditional sex toys. The remote-control feature allows partners to connect and share intimate moments no matter where they are, easing the pain of distance while enhancing excitement. The We-Vibe Sync can be controlled through the app, making it easy to use, personalise, and discreetly adjust during use.

The We-Vibe Sync is a perfect travel companion, being lightweight and discreet, with an included charging/storage case to keep things organised and charged on the go. It is also fully waterproof, meaning you can take your long-distance intimacy into the bath or shower.

The Sync is made from skin-friendly, body-safe silicone, making it hygienic, durable, and safe for use for everyone. Additionally, it is easy to clean and has multiple vibration speeds. In summary, the We-Vibe Sync stands out among other sex toys for long distance couples due to its versatility, convenience, and creativity.

Overall, the We-Vibe Sync is an excellent investment for long-distance couples who desire new, enjoyable ways to build intimacy. Its innovative design, coupled with the latest technology, ensures that partners can easily reach new heights of sexual pleasure and mutual satisfaction. It can be used for solo or duo play, making it multi-functional and flexible in its use.

Whether you are living in different parts of the world or separated due to circumstances, the We-Vibe Sync provides long-distance couples with a unique way to experience excitement, connection, and sexual fulfilment beyond distance. Being in control of each other's toys and pleasure, hearing the moans and groans and breathing in their ears also adds spice to heated moments.

In conclusion, the We-Vibe Sync is undoubtedly among the best sex toys for long distance relationships, providing couples with enhanced connectivity, intimacy, and fulfilment. Investing in the We-Vibe Sync is a wise choice for couples who seek to explore new and enjoyable ways to share intimacy no matter where they are. It brings a revolutionary approach to how sex toys can support long-distance relationships, providing an immersive and interactive experience that deepens emotional intimacy and enhances pleasure.

Moreover, the app-controlled feature of this sex toy provides couples with remote control capabilities, making it excellent for use in long-distance relationships. It is waterproof, travel-friendly, and made from hygienic materials, ensuring its durability and value for money.

In conclusion, the We-Vibe Sync offers one of the most promising and innovative solutions for couples seeking to enhance their sexual relationship through the use of technology. Whether for solo or duo play, it will undoubtedly serve you well as long as there's interest!

# Chapter 4

## OhMiBod BlueMotion Nex1

The OhMiBod BlueMotion Nex1 represents one of the most innovative sex toys for long-distance couples seeking to intensify their intimacy remotely. It is more than just a wearable vibrator; it offers a new level of sexual connectivity and stimulation between partners.

The device is a small wearable vibrator that can easily be placed inside a woman's underwear to stimulate both the clitoris and G-spot. It is controlled remotely via Bluetooth, allowing users to connect with one another from miles apart. The vibrator has five vibration features and patterns, adjustable through the app.

The OhMiBod BlueMotion Nex1 provides users with an immersive and interactive experience that brings unprecedented communication and interconnectivity during sex. By controlling your partner's pleasure, you build mutual trust and include diverse ways of self-love and care regardless of distance.

This sex toy is a great pick for long-distance couples because of its unique features and benefits. First and foremost, it allows couples to explore new realms of intimacy, despite being miles apart. The vibrations generated and controlled remotely through the app allow partners to stay incredibly close and build up intense orgasmic experiences.

The OhMiBod BlueMotion Nex1's compact and lightweight design means that it is discreet and easy to wear, making it great for public play or travel. Moreover, the device is USB rechargeable, so no need to worry about batteries or tangled cords.

The Bluetooth connectivity feature allows it to be effortlessly controlled while aside from each other, giving freedom and versatility to long-distance couples unable to enjoy sexual intimacy together more frequently. Another incredible bit of the vibrator is its adjustable vibration patterns, audible feedback and even touch screen capabilities.

Furthermore, the OhMiBod BlueMotion Nex1 promotes healthy communication and reinforces trust within a relationship. As couples explore their sexual desires and preferences, feedback about the device's intensities can be shared via app feedback or sound, allowing users to adjust the device settings and generate customized vibrations that suits their needs.

Best Sex Toys for Long Distance Relationship

For partners with limited opportunities for physical experiences together, the OhMiBod BlueMotion Nex1 offers a new level of sensual connection by building mutual anticipation, desire and pleasure through online control. It brings together the sensuality and pleasure of physical touch and technology and integrates into any long-distance couple's sexual routine.

In conclusion, The OhMiBod BlueMotion Nex1 stands as among the most impressive sex tech gadgets and is a top pick for couples in long-distance relationships. Its features and benefits go beyond the erotic- enhancing emotional connections and building trust, a great addition to any sexually explorative couple looking to push boundaries and explore exciting new realms of pleasures and intimacy. Whether couples are separated by distance or time commitments, this toy allows them to connect through mutual pleasure, building up intense levels of satisfaction and trust.

Ultimately, if you're in search of a high-quality sex toy that will elevate your online intimacy and relationships, the OhMiBod BlueMotion Nex1 offers premium quality, comfort, and superior innovation, making it an excellent tool for heightened pleasure and sexual exploration with a long-distance partner. So, bring the sense of touch closer to those you care the most with the BlueMotion Nex1.

# Chapter 5

## Lovense Max 2

The Lovense Max 2 is an exceptional male masturbator that is perfect for long-distance couples who want to experiment with mutual masturbation. It offers a fully interactive experience, allowing couples to connect and engage in intense pleasure from miles apart.

The device has an ergonomic design that accommodates the user's length and provides a comfortable and pleasurable experience. It also comes equipped with two air vents that allow users to adjust the pressure level, providing personalized pleasure levels. The Max 2 connects via Bluetooth and internet to Lovense's app, which allows for remote control by your partner, sound-activated features, and even having control through webcams.

One of the device's fantastic features is the ability to sync it with interactive adult content, ensuring that the vibration and suction automatically adjust to the corresponding sex scenes. Moreover, it offers a live video chat option between long-distance partners, providing an immersive and interactive experience that brings couples closer together, regardless of the distance.

The Lovense Max 2 is a great pick for long-distance couples for several reasons. Firstly, it allows couples to experience incredible pleasure together, even when they are miles apart. The connectivity feature means that you can control the device from anywhere in the world, as long as you have an internet connection.

Secondly, the Lovense Max 2 promotes communication and trust between partners, allowing them to share their sensuality remotely and create erotic experiences cumulatively. The app not only controls the device's vibration, but it also generates different touch sensations based on how fast or slow your partner interacts with LELO toy or engage with virtual content, building a symbolic routine to keep in touch and also providing feedback based on changes during use for better communication and trust.

Finally, the ease of use and convenience of the Lovense Max 2 makes it a top pick for long-distance couples who want to enhance their sexual experiences. The device is user-friendly, travel-friendly, discreet, and super easy to clean. It is also very quiet, allowing users to enjoy intimate moments without attracting unwanted attention.

The versatility of the Lovense Max 2 makes it stand out from other male masturbators on the market. It allows couples to connect in sexy and new ways; from syncing with adult content, sound activated settings or touch screen controls, as well as voice and video chat, the Max 2 encourages intimacy and experimentation, whether you are physically together or apart.

In summary, the Lovense Max 2 is a must-have for long-distance couples looking for new, fun, and exciting ways to be intimate with each other. The device's advanced features, easy-to-use interfaces, and interactive app opens up a realm of possibilities for mutual pleasure, which is essential in long-distance relationships. The Lovense Max 2 allows couples to explore their sensuality and sexuality in every way possible. It's another tool to add variety and spice up the love life of long distance couples.

The device is highly recommended, thanks to its innovative technology, connectivity features, versatility, and hassle-free design. It's perfect for those wanting to maintain intimacy in their long-distance relationship without sacrificing pleasure and fun.

In adding the Lovense Max 2 to one's intimate life as a long-distance couple, it can provide the desired sexual relief and expression that a relationship needs. Therefore, long-distance couples must invest in this wonderful toy for unparalleled pleasure, an intimate online experience, and a bond that will get stronger with each passing day.

# **Chapter 6**

## **Lovense Nora**

The Lovense Nora is a premium rabbit vibrator designed for long-distance couples. This vibrator has become increasingly popular thanks to its advanced technology features and its ability to connect couples across borders. The toy's functionality is optimized through the Lovense app, which adds more fun, excitement, and intimacy to the couple's sexual life.

The Lovense Nora Rabbit vibrator is easy and comfortable to use, making it a great choice for any level of experience. It has a curved shaft that massages the g-spot while its bunny ears stimulate the clitoris. Apart from the traditional vibration modes, the Nora provides customizable settings like rotating tip patterns and vibrations levels based on the user's preference.

The Lovense Nora's primary purpose is to offer an interactive, immersive sexual experience for couples separated by distance. Partners can control the device via the Lovenes app, actively engaging in each other's intimate moments. The app exploits technology and allows couples to integrate long-distance intimacy into their relationship by modifying a toy's setting, touching, sound, or webcam, expanding horizons for LDR couples' sex lives. Couples can explore different settings and experiment with each other to create an ultimate experience unique to their preferences.

One of the advantages of using the Lovense Nora rabbit vibrator is its ability to stimulate the pleasure points in both partners remotely, adding more intimacy even from miles apart. With internet connectivity, the Lovense Nora enables couples to interact regardless of any geographical distance, keeping the love and spark alive in their sex life.

Additionally, Lovense Nora's design is ergonomic, providing comfort and versatility in use, adding more depth to the user's experience. The vibrator is also completely waterproof, making it perfect for seamless usage during shower activities.

The Lovense Nora is an exceptional pick for couples in long-distance relationships for several reasons. Firstly, it's an interactive toy that allows partners to control its various functions remotely. The app's easy-to-use interface can be used on both iOS and Android devices, allowing couples to connect and use the product from anywhere.

Secondly, the Lovense Nora is designed to create a personalized experience for each individual user that can be easily modified according to their preferences. Additionally, the Lovense app provides features such as video calls, texting options, and a control screen to make the experience more interactive and customizable.

Thirdly, the Lovense Nora highlights the importance of intimacy and connection in a long-distance relationship, becoming an instrument to bridge that physical distance gap. The product encourages open communication and experimentation between couples, which strengthens trust and emotional bonds ultimately resulting in a more fulfilling sexual life.

In conclusion, the Lovense Nora is the perfect sex toy for couples in a long-distance relationship who want to maintain intimacy and explore their sexuality and sexual boundaries. The product's versatile design, combined with the interactive Lovense app, offers couples a range of functions for optimum pleasure.

The Lovense Nora satisfies clitoral and g-spot stimulation in a unique way through its bunny ear and curved tip design. Combined with the intelligent rotating function in its shaft, the Lovense Nora delivers a powerful crescendo of orgasms.

Long-distance couples no longer have to compromise pleasure or intimacy due to distance. With Lovense Nora, couples can enjoy fulfilling sexual experiences that will keep them connected despite the miles between them. The Lovense Nora is an ideal pick for any couple looking to spice up their sex life with painless customization to tailor to individual preferences and redefine their sexual experience.

# Chapter 7

## We-Vibe Moxie

The We-Vibe Moxie is a small and discreet wearable vibrator specifically designed for long-distance couples looking to spice up their intimacy. It's a unique adult product that offers both clitoral and g-spot stimulation with its precise, angled design, ensuring maximum pleasure.

The We-Vibe Moxie's primary function is to offer hands-free pleasure that delicately rubs the clitoris while having sex or performing daily chores. The wearable vibrator offers powerful vibrations for discreet public usage, allowing couples to enjoy intimacy wherever and whenever they choose, creating moments of spontaneous fun and passion.

The device is easy to use and comes with a remote that gives you control over the vibration patterns and intensity, providing a customizable experience based on the user's preference. The vibrating panty-integrated We-Vibe Moxie allows men to wear it on their penis, increasing the quality and efficiency of penetrative sex as the vibrations stimulate both the clitoris and penis simultaneously, creating a heightened sexual experience for both partners.

The We-Vibe Moxie is a great pick for long-distance couples because of its unique design and various usage possibilities. The device's wearable nature allows couples to integrate it into their daily lives, no matter how busy or far apart they are. With the remote control, the device is perfect for interactive sessions where partners can take control of each other's pleasure.

Moreover, the We-Vibe Moxie offers unparalleled discretion, making it ideal for couples who want to have fun and explore their sexual boundaries in public places discreetly. Couples can use the vibrator in public areas or video calls, adding more excitement and intimacy to their sexual lives.

Additionally, the We-Vibe Moxie is compact and lightweight, making it portable, easy to clean, and comfortable to wear. It can be discreetly tucked away in a purse or bag for on-the-go usage when needed. Its whisper-quiet motor ensures that you're the only ones who know about your little secret, allowing you to enjoy sexual pleasure anywhere you may go - without worrying about noise levels.

Furthermore, the We-Vibe Moxie is made with high-quality materials that are body-safe and hypoallergenic, ensuring its safety and long-lasting use. The device's design contours to the natural shape of your body, making it comfortable to wear for extended periods, while still offering powerful vibrations that deliver intense orgasms every time.

Overall, the We-Vibe Moxie is an excellent pick for long-distance couples looking for a discreet and portable device that enhances intimacy, allows customization, and offers hands-free stimulation. The device's unique features and design make it a perfect sex toy for couples who are far apart but still want to maintain their sexual connection. Whether using it for interactive sessions or introducing some fun into your daily life, the We-Vibe Moxie can transform how long-distance couples experience pleasure.

By creating new possibilities and opportunities for exploring your sexual desires, the We-Vibe Moxie offers a unique form of intimacy that brings couples closer together despite the physical distance. The device's vibration patterns and intensity levels allow for customizations, providing you with a personalized experience that enhances your sexual pleasure and helps you achieve mind-blowing orgasms.

As couples navigate the challenges of maintaining a fulfilling sexual relationship while being apart, the We-Vibe Moxie stands out as an affordable and efficient solution to keep the sexual spark alive. It is an ideal sex toy for long-distance couples who are looking for ways to enhance their intimacy while being miles apart. So, if you are in a long-distance relationship and looking for something to help maintain that connection, the We-Vibe Moxie could be the perfect addition to your virtual romance toolkit.

In summary, the We-Vibe Moxie is a discreet and wearable vibrator that provides hands-free pleasure through both clitoral and g-spot stimulation. It comes with a remote control that allows users to customize the device's vibration patterns and intensity. The product's body-safe materials, comfortable design, customizable options, and discretion make it an ideal pick for long-distance couples looking to enhance their intimacy and explore their sexuality.

# Chapter 8

## Kiiroo Titan Interactive Vibrating Stroker

The Kiiroo Titan Interactive Vibrating Stroker is a high-tech male masturbation device that can be used either on its own or as part of the Kiiroo Onyx+ Pearl2 Couples Set, making it an excellent pick for long-distance couples looking to explore their sexual desires.

The device's main function is to offer hands-free pleasure to men by creating a realistic stimulation feel that emulates real penetrative intercourse. The vibrating stroker has an interactive system that responds to movement, making it perfect for a solo user or as part of long-distance intimacy. Additionally, the device is equipped with a series of motors that can be customized to particular vibration patterns and intensity levels using the Kiiroo app.

The Kiiroo Titan Interactive Vibrating Stroker is the perfect pick for long-distance couples because it allows for distance and time to exist between partners while maintaining their sexual connection. The device is compatible with other Kiiroo products, allowing couples to sync their devices remotely through a mobile app and experience interactive sex in real-time. This synchronization feature enables couples to create their own intimate sessions, despite being miles apart. Partners can also control the stroker's vibration levels remotely, adding excitement and pleasure to their virtual intimacy.

Another reason that makes the Kiiroo Titan Interactive Vibrating Stroker an excellent choice for long-distance couples is its user-friendly design. The stroker is ergonomically designed to fit comfortably in hand, ensuring users have a comfortable grip during use. Its lightweight and compact size make it ideal for transportation, allowing you to take your sexual pleasure wherever you go.

Moreover, the device is made with high-quality silicone, ensuring its durability and safety while being hypoallergenic and easy to clean.

In terms of use, the Kiiroo Titan Interactive Vibrating Stroker works by sliding your penis inside the device where the powerful motors take over to provide pleasurable vibrations. The device also has a pressure-sensitive pad on the exterior that responds to the movements you make, creating an interactive and personalized experience.

The stroker has nine vibration modes that offer various levels of intensity, allowing users to customize their experience to their preferences. The Kiiroo mobile app complements the device, giving you even more control over the experience. Through the app, you can choose from an extensive library of interactive videos, sync partner devices, and explore partner pleasure maps, paving the way for an immersive and interactive sexual experience.

Overall, the Kiiroo Titan Interactive Vibrating Stroker is a fantastic pick for long-distance couples looking to enhance their intimacy. Its interactive system, customizable vibration modes, and compatibility with other Kiiroo products including the Onyx+ Pearl2 Couples Set make the device a standout option. The real-time synchronization features allow couples to explore new sexual possibilities remotely ensuring they can be present for each other in times of physical distance.

Whether you use it as an interactive toy with your partner or as a solo pleasure tool, the Kiiroo Titan Interactive Vibrating Stroker is flexible enough to satisfy all your fantasies. Its sleek design and body-safe silicone make it easy and safe to clean, while it's compact size fits comfortably in hand, making it ideal for travel.

In conclusion, the Kiiroo Titan Interactive Vibrating Stroker is a highly recommended sex toy for long-distance couples who want to keep the passion alive despite being miles apart. It gives couples the opportunity to explore each other's sexuality in new ways, and can help create intimacy in the virtual realm. The device's innovative design, combined with its customizable settings and interactive features, offer a truly unique and personalized experience that is difficult to find with traditional masturbators.

Couples can enhance their pleasure and take their relationship to the next level with this revolutionary sex toy. Whether you are spending time apart or simply looking for new ways to enhance your sexual play, the Kiiroo Titan Interactive Vibrating Stroker is an ideal addition to your adult toy collection. With this device, couples can bring some diversity and excitement to their intimate moments, ensuring they keeping the flame of passion burning bright, even when distance separates them.

# Chapter 9

## Je Joue Dua Vibrating Kegel Balls

Je Joue Dua Vibrating Kegel Balls are high-quality and sleek kegel balls that offer women an excellent way to enhance their pleasure and strengthen their pelvic muscles. These balls have quickly become popular among women seeking to improve their sexual health and performance while having a blast.

The main function of the Je Joue Dua Vibrating Kegel Balls is to strengthen the pelvic muscles by providing resistance during exercises. The device comes with two weighted balls that can be inserted into the vagina, which then allows women to strengthen their muscles by clamping down and holding the balls in place. This process helps to tone and tighten the pelvic floor muscles, leading to better bladder control, prevention of uterine prolapse, and improving sexual function.

The Je Joue Dua Vibrating Kegel Ballsare also designed for intimate play and sexual pleasure. The device also comes with an accompanying remote control that allows you to switch between its 10 different vibration settings and intensities. The remote control can be used to set the vibration modes and intensities, which can be adapted to your individual preferences. The device is perfect for solo play or during lovemaking, adding an extra level of pleasure and sensation to your intimate experiences.

For those in long-distance relationships, the Je Joue Dua Vibrating Kegel Balls are an excellent choice as they come equipped with a connectivity feature that allows couples to control each other's vibrational plays through the Je Joue app. This added feature makes it easier for couples to connect and engage during intimate moments despite being separated by miles. It offers an exciting opportunity for couples to tease and tantalize each other from afar, enhancing their sexual connection even when they are miles apart.

What sets the Je Joue Dua Vibrating Kegel Balls apart from other kegel balls on the market is its unique and advanced technology. The design of these balls is such that they can be programmed to vibrate with millions of different patterns. These patterns can be adapted by the user to create entirely new pulsing experiences, which can be shared with partners who are far away through the Je Joue app.

Moreover, the Je Joue Dua Vibrating Kegel Balls are made of high-quality silicone, which is body-safe, hypoallergenic, and easy-to-clean. They are also rechargeable and have a long-lasting battery life that can provide hours of playtime with just one charge. The balls are compact and discreet, making them ideal for travel, and the accompanying remote control offers seamless control over the device's functions.

In conclusion, the Je Joue Dua Vibrating Kegel Balls are the ultimate kegel balls, designed to enhance your sexual pleasure, improve your pelvic health, and provide couples with a unique way to bond despite long distances. Its connectivity feature allows couples to experience intimate moments together through their smart devices, making it easier to maintain emotional and sexual intimacy even when physically apart.

These innovative Kegel balls provide users with an excellent option for toning and strengthening their pelvic muscles, and its advanced technology enables users to try out new and exciting pulsing sensations. Additionally, its compact and discreet design make it easy to take everywhere you go. This device offers women a comprehensive tool for enhancing their sexual and reproductive health, and aids in building a stronger and more fulfilling relationship with their partner. Overall, the Je Joue Dau Vibrating Kegel Balls is an excellent choice for women who enjoy keeping in touch with their partner and maintaining intimacy despite distance. With this device, couples can explore new levels of pleasure, spice up their intimate moments, and achieve the ultimate satisfaction they have always desired. The Je Joue Dua Vibrating Kegel Balls are just one of the many sex toys in the market designed to help couples maintain intimacy despite distance, and with the rise of technology and innovative designs, couples no longer need to feel disconnected when they are miles apart.

# Chapter 10

## Womanizer Premium Clitoral Stimulator

The Womanizer Premium Clitoral Stimulator is one of the most popular adult sex toys that drive every woman to experience the ultimate orgasm. It is a powerful sex toy that uses patented Pleasure Air Technology and 12 intense levels of stimulation to provide an unprecedented level of pleasure that users can't help but crave more of.

When it comes to sex, distance shouldn't be a hindrance to the amount of pleasure you can get. With Womanizer Premium Clitoral Stimulator, you and your partner can enjoy full stimulation that surpasses physical obstacles without being physically present with each other.

The stimulator's use is straightforward; you only need to place the nozzle over your clit and let the toy handle the rest. The suction and pressure waves work to enhance blood flow to your intimate area, and this leads to incredible waves of pleasure. The Womanizer comes with replaceable silicone stimulation heads that provide full comfort during use and make it perfect for long distance couples.

One of the significant advantages of the Womanizer Premium Clitoral Stimulator is its seamless connectivity capabilities. This toy features a Smart Silence technology that ensures that it only turns on when it is in place. Couple this with its Bluetooth connectivity, and it becomes very easy to control the toy from across the room or even miles away from each other.

The Womanizer is an excellent pick for long-distance couples because it offers unlimited possibilities for both partners. For one, it allows one partner to experience the sensation and pleasure involved with the same intensity as if they were both together at the same time. It is also perfect for adding some excitement and variety to your long-distance sessions.

With its different stimulation levels, modes, and patterns, you can explore and experiment with new ways to experience pleasurable sensations, which keeps things fresh and exciting for your long-distance relationship.

The Womanizer Premium Clitoral Stimulator is an exceptional adult sex toy that offers a seamless and thrilling sexual experience for long-distance couples. It's easy to use, comfortable, and provides unlimited possibilities for both partners involved. If you're in a long-distance relationship and are in need of a high-quality, versatile, and efficient sex toy, then the Womanizer Premium Clitoral Stimulator is an excellent choice for you and your partner.

# Chapter 11

## Lovense Hush

The Lovense Hush is a powerful, high-tech butt plug designed to give users the ultimate pleasure, even when they are miles away from each other. This sex toy offers both partners an intense and enjoyable experience that translates to an incredible sense of intimacy in a long-distance relationship.

The Lovense Hush is made from body-safe silicone material with an insertable length of up to 3.94 inches. The base of the butt plug features an excellent size and shape that provides full support and ease of use during the play. It also comes with a comfortable and adjustable neck that offers the perfect fit while ensuring that the toy stays securely in place during use.

The Hush is specifically designed for remote control, meaning your partner can control the device or vibrations via the Lovense app from anywhere, allowing for a hands-free sex toy experience. This is perfect for long-distance couples who want to enjoy fun and intimate playtime together in spite of the distance between them.

The Lovense Hush is perfect for long-distance couples because it offers unlimited possibilities. With its app control functionality, users can play with the various vibration modes, or customize their own patterns to suit their preferences. The remote control feature allows partners to interact with each other and create a unique and exciting sexual stimulation that goes beyond what is possible through text or video calls.

Also, the Lovense Hush offers exclusive features like "Sound Activated Vibrations" which are excellent for interactive sessions during groovy music or naughty whispers. It also provides carefree control options like touch-screen vibration control, alternative Wi-Fi connectivity, and many more.

In conclusion, the Lovense Hush is an exceptional sex toy that offers seamless, hands-free pleasure for long-distance couples. The app control feature makes it perfect for partners looking to build more intimacy and excitement into their relationships, whilst providing an intensely pleasurable experience with the different vibration modes and abilities to customize the stimulation patterns.

So, if you're in a long-distance relationship and searching for an effective, high-quality and versatile sex toy, then the Lovense Hush is undoubtedly worth considering as your first pick.

# Chapter 12

## Lelo Hugo Prostate Massager

The Lelo Hugo Prostate Massager is a high-tech and luxurious sex toy designed for men who want to experience the ultimate pleasure, both alone or with their partners. It is an incredible device specially made to stimulate the prostate gland, located next to the rectum and known to be one of the primary sources of male sexual pleasure.

The device features dual motors - one for prostate stimulation and the other for perineum stimulation, providing men with a mind-blowing combination of sensations. At Lelo Hugo's base, it has a comfortable handle that is easy to control, and the rounded tip provides easy penetration.

One of the great features of the device is its app control, which enables long-distance couples to play together no matter how far apart they might be physically. With Lelo's innovative SenseMotion technology, you can explore a myriad of vibration patterns, ranging from gentle to intense, depending on your solo or couple's needs and preferences.

The Lelo Hugo Prostate Massager is a fantastic toy for long-distance couples because it puts control in their hands. With the app control functionality, both partners can take turns controlling the device, creating customized vibrations, and exploring new and exciting sensations. This enables couples to experience more intimate and pleasurable moments even when they are miles apart from each other.

Apart from having app control, the Lelo Hugo is made of body-safe materials that are comfortable, hygienic, and easy to clean. It is also rechargeable, water-resistant, and comes with a travel lock, making it perfect for journeys and discreet storage.

In conclusion, the Lelo Hugo Prostate Massager is a brilliant sex toy for men looking to explore their sexuality, especially in long-distance relationships. With its unique SenseMotion technology and dual motors, this device will not only help men achieve powerful orgasms but also help couples explore new levels of intimacy and pleasure from far away. Its app control feature makes it simple and easy to use, providing limitless possibilities to customize different stimulation modes, intensities, and patterns. Therefore, the Lelo Hugo is undoubtedly one of the best options for long-distance couples looking for a high-quality and effective prostate massager.

# Chapter 13

## Lovense Ambi Bullet Vibrator

The Lovense Ambi Bullet Vibrator is a dynamic and interactive sex toy that sexes up your solo and couple's playtime. It is a small, egg-shaped vibrator designed with unique triangular asymmetry, which means it can be comfortably used as both an internal or external vibrator. This feature provides users with a wide range of stimulation options to explore.

The device uses Bluetooth and the latest Lovense app, which enables users to interact and play together, even from different physical locations. At home or away, controlling the vibrators is simple and opens up a world of possibilities, thanks to the app's rich features.

Long-distance partners can take turns controlling the vibration intensity, pattern, and rhythm using the app's virtual control panel. The app allows users to store previously used settings for the Lovense Ambi, which makes it comfortable to switch between them without missing your preferred modes.

The Lovense Ambi Bullet Vibrator is a great pick for long-distance couples since its compact and travel-friendly design makes it an excellent choice for discreet playtime during virtual dates or personal sessions. Its unique triangular shape means it can be tucked away comfortably in your panties without anyone noticing. This feature was specifically designed for women who love hands-free stimulation during long-distance playtime.

In addition, the Lovense Ambi is made of body-safe silicone material that is both easy to clean and hygienic. It is also rechargeable, and a single charge provides up to 3 hours of playing time. The Lovense Ambi is water-resistant, making it perfect for use in the shower, bathtub, or pool.

To sum up, the Lovense Ambi Bullet Vibrator is an excellent sex toy for couples in long-distance relationships. It is perfect for taking your intimate moments to the next level, allowing you to explore different vibration patterns, intensities, and rhythms remotely using the Lovense app. The device's unique triangular shape is comfortable and provides users with a range of stimulation options. Furthermore, it is compact, easy to store, and travel-friendly, making it perfect for discreet playtime on-the-go.

Cheryl Bach

# Chapter 14

## We-Vibe Verge

The We-Vibe Verge is an innovative vibrating gadget designed for penis owners looking to enhance their pleasure levels. It's a silicone cock ring that vibrates around the base of the penis while also providing gentle pressure on the perineum (the area between the anus and scrotum). This device is entirely flexible, allowing you to adjust the pressure and intensity according to your preference.

The We-Vibe Verge is perfect for both solo and couple's playtime - it's a great way to explore different sensations and take your sex life to new heights. With its powerful and quiet motor, the We-Vibe Verge generates deep and rumbly vibrations that can be felt throughout the entire body.

Long-distance couples will find this device especially appealing due to its app-controlled feature. Once downloaded, the We-Connect app allows couples to explore and enjoy each other from any distance. With the app, you can create custom vibration patterns and play with one another even when you're miles apart. Couples can trade control of the device, creating a heightened sense of intimacy and allowing for mutual stimulation.

The We-Vibe Verge is a fantastic pick for long-distance couples because it adds an exciting level of interactivity to their relationship. Couples can use the device to help bridge the gap between them and maintain their sexual connection while they're apart. The app is easy to use, which means you don't need to be tech-savvy to get started.

Moreover, the We-Vibe Verge is made of medical-grade silicone material, which makes it both body-safe and hygienic. It's rechargeable, waterproof, easy to clean, and provides up to two hours of uninterrupted playtime. Additionally, the We-Vibe Verge is designed to be both comfortable and secure, providing you with a snug fit during use.

In conclusion, if you're looking for a sex toy that can enhance intimacy and pleasure between long-distance couples, then the We-Vibe Verge is an excellent option to consider. Its app-controlled feature is perfect for couples looking to stay connected while they're apart, and its powerful motor and comfortable design make it an enjoyable sex toy for solo playtime too. The device is body-safe, rechargeable, waterproof, easy to use and clean, and provides users with up to two hours of playtime.

# Chapter 15

## Kiiroo Cliona

The Kiiroo Cliona is a sleek and stylish sex toy designed for women who are looking to experience hands-free orgasms. It's a clitoral vibrator that uses air pressure technology to deliver waves of pleasure to the clitoris. The device is made of medical-grade silicone material and features an ergonomic design for a comfortable and secure fit during use.

The Kiiroo Cliona is perfect for solo playtime and can also be used by long-distance couples to enhance their intimacy and pleasure. Using the Kiiroo app, couples can connect with one another via Bluetooth and Wi-Fi, allowing them to control each other's device from anywhere in the world. The app allows you to create custom vibration patterns and explore different sensations, turning your virtual interactions into exciting and explosive moments of pleasure.

The Kiiroo Cliona is a fantastic pick for long distance couples because it offers a level of interactivity and intimacy that is hard to match with other sex toys. With the app, couples can create personalized vibration patterns, share intimate moments, and even make video calls while experiencing synchronized sensations, making it an excellent tool for maintaining sexual connections.

Furthermore, the Kiiroo Cliona is rechargeable and waterproof, making it perfect for use in the bath or shower. It has an ultra-quiet motor, which means you can enjoy discreet playtime without worrying about anyone hearing it. The device is lightweight and portable, allowing you to take it with you wherever you go, making it ideal for adventurous couples who like to spice things up on-the-go.

In conclusion, if you're looking for a hands-free clitoral vibrator that can enhance intimacy and pleasure between long-distance couples, then the Kiiroo Cliona is an excellent option to consider. Its sleek and stylish design, air pressure technology, and app-controlled feature make it perfect for solo playtime and virtual interaction with your partner. The device is also made of medical-grade silicone material, rechargeable, waterproof, and lightweight, allowing you to take it with you wherever you go. The Kiiroo Cliona is definitely a great addition to any couple's sex toy collection!

Cheryl Bach

# Chapter 16

## Fleshlight Launch

The Fleshlight Launch is an innovative male sex toy designed to enhance pleasure during solo playtime for men. It's a high-tech masturbator that allows men to experience an extremely realistic sexual experience with its automated stroking mechanism. The device is made of premium materials, mimicking the feel and texture of real skin, and features a luxury design.

The Fleshlight Launch is perfect for solo play and can also be used by long-distance couples, especially those in long-distance relationships, to enhance intimacy and pleasure. Using the Kiiroo app or other compatible sex tech devices, couples can connect with each other via Bluetooth and Wi-Fi, allowing them to control the movements of the

Fleshlight Launch from anywhere in the world. This exciting feature allows couples to engage in virtual sexual interaction that feels incredibly realistic, making it a great pick for long distance couples who want to maintain their connection and intimacy.

In addition to its automated stroking mechanism and app-controlled feature, the Fleshlight Launch also has several other features that make it an excellent pick for men looking to enhance their solo play. The device allows you to adjust the length and speed of your strokes, allowing for a completely customizable experience that caters to personal preferences. Furthermore, the device is rechargeable and can provide up to two hours of uninterrupted playtime on a single charge.

The Fleshlight Launch is also compatible with a wide range of Fleshlight sleeves, providing a variety of sensations and textures to choose from, ensuring that your experience is never dull or tedious.

In conclusion, if you're a man seeking an interactive, high-tech masturbator that can enhance your solo play, the Fleshlight Launch is a great choice to consider. Not only does it provide an incredibly realistic sensation, but its app-controlled feature and adjustable stroking speed allows for a fully customizable experience. Moreover, the fact that it's rechargeable, compatible with a wide range of Fleshlight sleeves, and has a luxury design, makes it an excellent addition to any man's sex toy collection. And for long-distance couples, the Fleshlight Launch offers an intimate and interactive experience that can bring couples closer together, no matter where they are in the world. It's definitely a must-have sex toy for anyone seeking a new level of solo play pleasure or looking to enhance their long-distance relationship.

Cheryl Bach

# Chapter 17

## OhMiBod Esca 2

The OhMiBod Esca 2 is a powerful and versatile sex toy specially designed for women. It is a wearable G-spot vibrator that can be controlled through a smartphone app or a partner's device, making it an ideal tool for long-distance couples who want to maintain intimacy and pleasure. The device is made of body-safe silicone, which is soft, hypoallergenic, and easy to clean.

Designed with a wireless Bluetooth connection, this vibrator has a built-in LED indicator that alerts you to incoming messages, so you never miss out on anything important. The OhMiBod Esca 2 also features powerful motors that deliver intense vibrations directly to the G-spot, providing incredible stimulation that leads to intense orgasms.

The device is easy to use and set up, even for beginners. The OhMiBod Esca 2 can be controlled via the OhMiBod Remote app, available for both iOS and Android, which allows you to control the intensity of the vibrations manually or through pre-set patterns. The app also features a messaging system, allowing you to exchange messages and emoticons with your partner while controlling the vibrator.

One of the best things about the OhMiBod Esca 2 is its size and shape; it's small enough to be discreet and easy to wear, making it an excellent option to use in public places without drawing attention. Furthermore, the device's rechargeable battery lasts up to three hours and is USB chargeable, giving you freedom from having to replace batteries frequently.

Best Sex Toys for Long Distance Relationship

For long-distance couples in particular, the OhMiBod Esca 2 is an excellent choice, enabling couples to experience pleasure and intimacy even when miles apart. The app-controlled feature allows partners to connect and interact in real-time, making the distance between them feel much shorter. The device is designed with discrete vibrations, making it an ideal and safe option during public use, making it perfect for couples who enjoy spicing things up in adventurous locations.

The OhMiBod Esca 2 will undoubtedly kick your sex toy collection up a notch, providing unprecedented levels of thrill and stimulation that can drive both you and your partner wild. Its wearable design, app-controlled feature, and powerful motors make it one of the best sex toys on the market, and a must-have for long-distance couples seeking an intimate and interactive sexual experience.

Cheryl Bach

# Chapter 18

## We-Vibe Chorus

We-Vibe Chorus is a versatile and innovative adult sex toy that is perfect for long distance couples. It's a wearable vibrator that is designed to stimulate both partners simultaneously, whether they are in the same location or miles apart.

The We-Vibe Chorus can be used in a variety of ways and positions. It's one of the best sex toy choices for long distance couples because it comes equipped with a mobile app that allows partners to control the toy from their smartphones, regardless of their location.

This device is designed with high-quality silicone material, ensuring that it's safe for both partners and easy to clean. With its adjustable fit, the We-Vibe Chorus is comfortable for both partners to wear for extended periods of time. Its dual-stimulation design targets both the clitoris and G-spot, providing intense and pleasurable sensations. The vibrator is not overly loud, so it's a great choice for discreet use in public or shared living spaces.

Long distance couples will appreciate the We-Vibe Chorus' remote control and mobile app features, which give them both an added level of intimacy even when they're apart. The app allows partners to control the toy through a secure Bluetooth connection, and offers plenty of customization options for vibration patterns and strengths.

The We-Vibe Chorus is a great pick for long distance couples because it helps them feel more connected and close despite the distance between them. With its convenient mobile app and dual-stimulation design, both partners can experience pleasure and intimacy together, no matter where they are.

Overall, the We-Vibe Chorus is an excellent choice for couples looking to enhance their long distance relationships with the added intimacy and pleasure of a wearable vibrator. Whether you're in a long distance relationship, or just looking for new ways to explore and enjoy your sexuality together, the We-Vibe Chorus provides an unforgettable experience that both partners will appreciate.

So, if you're looking for a discreet, versatile, and innovative sex toy that can bring you and your partner closer together, then consider investing in the We-Vibe Chorus. With its advanced features and ergonomic design, it's definitely one of the best sex toys for long distance relationships out there!

Cheryl Bach

# Chapter 19

## Lelo Tiani 3

The Lelo Tiani 3 is a multi-functional, remote-controlled vibrator designed for couples. It's an advanced sex toy that can be used in a variety of ways to enhance sexual pleasure and intimacy.

The Lelo Tiani 3 is a wearable vibrator that stimulates both partners during sex. Its flexible design adjusts to fit the female anatomy comfortably and discreetly, allowing for hands-free use and ultimate versatility. The powerful motor provides intense vibrations to both the G-spot and clitoris, creating a truly unforgettable experience.

This sex toy comes with a compact remote control that allows partners to easily adjust the vibration patterns and intensities, even from long distances. The remote control gives long distance couples the ability to experience mutual pleasure and intimacy, no matter where they are.

The Lelo Tiani 3 is also waterproof, making it perfect for use in the shower or bath, and its rechargeable battery ensures long-lasting pleasure.

What makes the Lelo Tiani 3 an excellent pick for long distance couples is its ability to connect to the internet and be controlled using the We-Connect app. Once partners download the app on their smartphones and sign in to their shared We-Connect account, they can control and customize the vibrator's settings from anywhere in the world.

The app not only allows partners to synchronize their movements and vibrations, but it also provides added features like voice or video calls and chat capabilities, bringing a whole new level of intimacy to your long distance relationship.

In conclusion, the Lelo Tiani 3 is definitely one of the best sex toys for long distance couples. Its innovative design, powerful vibrations, and user-friendly features make it a great choice for anyone looking to enhance their connection with their partner no matter the distance. The remote control and smartphone app add an extra level of convenience, allowing couples to experience pleasure and intimacy together even when they can't physically be together.

The Lelo Tiani 3 also has a beautiful and ergonomic design, making it attractive and sensual to use both alone and with a partner. It provides hands-free stimulation during sex, leaving both partners' hands free to explore each other in other ways.

Thus, if you're looking to take your long-distance relationship to a new level of intimacy and pleasure, consider investing in the Lelo Tiani 3. With its advanced features and truly unforgettable sensations, it's one of the best choices for couples who want to stay intimately connected despite the distance between them.

# Chapter 20

## Lovense Edge

The Lovense Edge is a premium quality, adjustable prostate massager designed for men. It's an advanced sex toy that can help men achieve mind-blowing orgasms, even from a long distance.

The Lovense Edge is a wearable sex toy that stimulates the male prostate and perineum simultaneously. Its versatile design allows for easy customization to fit any anatomy comfortably and discreetly. The powerful motor provides strong and precise vibrations to those erogenous zones, creating a truly unforgettable experience.

This sex toy comes with a compact remote control that allows partners to easily adjust the vibration patterns and intensities, even from long distances. It also has a smartphone compatible app that enables real-time control, syncing with your favourite erotic content and offers unique features like sound-activated vibrations and long-distance control.

What makes the Lovense Edge an excellent pick for long distance couples is its ability to connect to the internet, allowing it to be controlled remotely from anywhere in the world. Once partners download the app and sign in to their shared Lovense account, they can control and customize the vibrator's settings. This means that regardless of whether you're in different countries or even on different continents, the Lovense Edge can bring you and your partner together in an intimate and pleasurable experience.

The Lovense Edge has a sleek and compact design, making it easy to carry and use discreetly. It is also made of soft and flexible silicone material, making it comfortable to use for an extended period.

Overall, the Lovense Edge is a fantastic sex toy for long distance couples who want to experiment with prostate stimulation and explore new levels of pleasure. Its user-friendly features, remote control, and sync-compatible app make it an excellent pick for couples looking to maintain intimacy and explore their sexuality despite the miles between them. The Lovense Edge is also waterproof, making it perfect for use in the shower or the bath.

The app not only allows couples to control and customize the Lovense Edge's settings, but it also adds new levels of excitement to the experience. Partners can chat with one another using the app, share erotic content, and even synchronize their orgasms, regardless of the distance.

The Lovense Edge is great for long distance couples because it allows you to get intimate whenever you want, wherever you are. With this sex toy, there are no limits to how you can please each other or enjoy pleasure together. It's a discreet and innovative addition to any couple's long distance toolkit and can revolutionize your intimacy.

To sum up, if you're looking for an advanced prostate massager that can help you achieve mind-blowing orgasms and maintain intimacy in your long-distance relationship, then the Lovense Edge is an excellent choice. Its wearable design, powerful vibrations, and remote control capability make it a fantastic pick for couples who are separated by distance. Moreover, the app-compatible technology adds new features and excitement to the experience, making it feel like you're right there with your partner. So, invest in Lovense Edge today for a revolutionary experience and enhance your long-distance sexual relationship.

# Conclusion

In conclusion, "Best Sex Toys for Long Distance Relationships: 20+ Top Adult Sex Toys for Long Distance Couples – Vibrators, Dildos, and Accessories" is a must-have guide for anyone in a long distance relationship who wants to keep their love life thrilling and satisfying.

By providing you with a thorough overview of the best sex toys available for long distance couples, this book can help you explore new levels of pleasure with your partner no matter where you are in the world. The recommendations provided in this book will not only help you choose the right toys for your unique needs but also educate you on effective ways to enhance your connection with your partner.

Cheryl Bach

Long distance relationships can be challenging, but investing in the right sex toys can make all the difference. With the expert guidance provided in this book, you'll be on your way to deeper intimacy and shared satisfaction.

So why wait? Start exploring the world of adult toys today and take your long distance relationship to new heights of pleasure and intimacy! Whether you're a seasoned pro when it comes to sex toys or a newbie looking to explore for the first time, this book has something for everyone. With "Best Sex Toys for Long Distance Relationships", you're sure to find the perfect additions to your intimate arsenal.

Remember, distance should never be a barrier to physical and emotional intimacy in your relationship. With the right tools and ongoing communication, long distance couples can still maintain a healthy and satisfying love life. This book is an invaluable resource that will help you achieve just that.

Invest in your intimacy and connection today with "Best Sex Toys for Long Distance Relationships: 20+ Top Adult Sex Toys for Long Distance Couples – Vibrators, Dildos, and Accessories".

Cheryl Bach